Your Colors

Written by: Mariah J. Tolson

Illustrations by: Marissa Nelson

Your Colors

Copyright © 2021 Mariah J. Tolson.

All rights reserved.

Welcome to Your Colors,

This book was written to inspire life into your wonderful child. It is filled with words of affirmations, and yoga to get your and your child's chakras aligned. I encourage you to, interact and engage with the movements while you read so that we all shine together!

Peace and Love

Mariah J Tolson

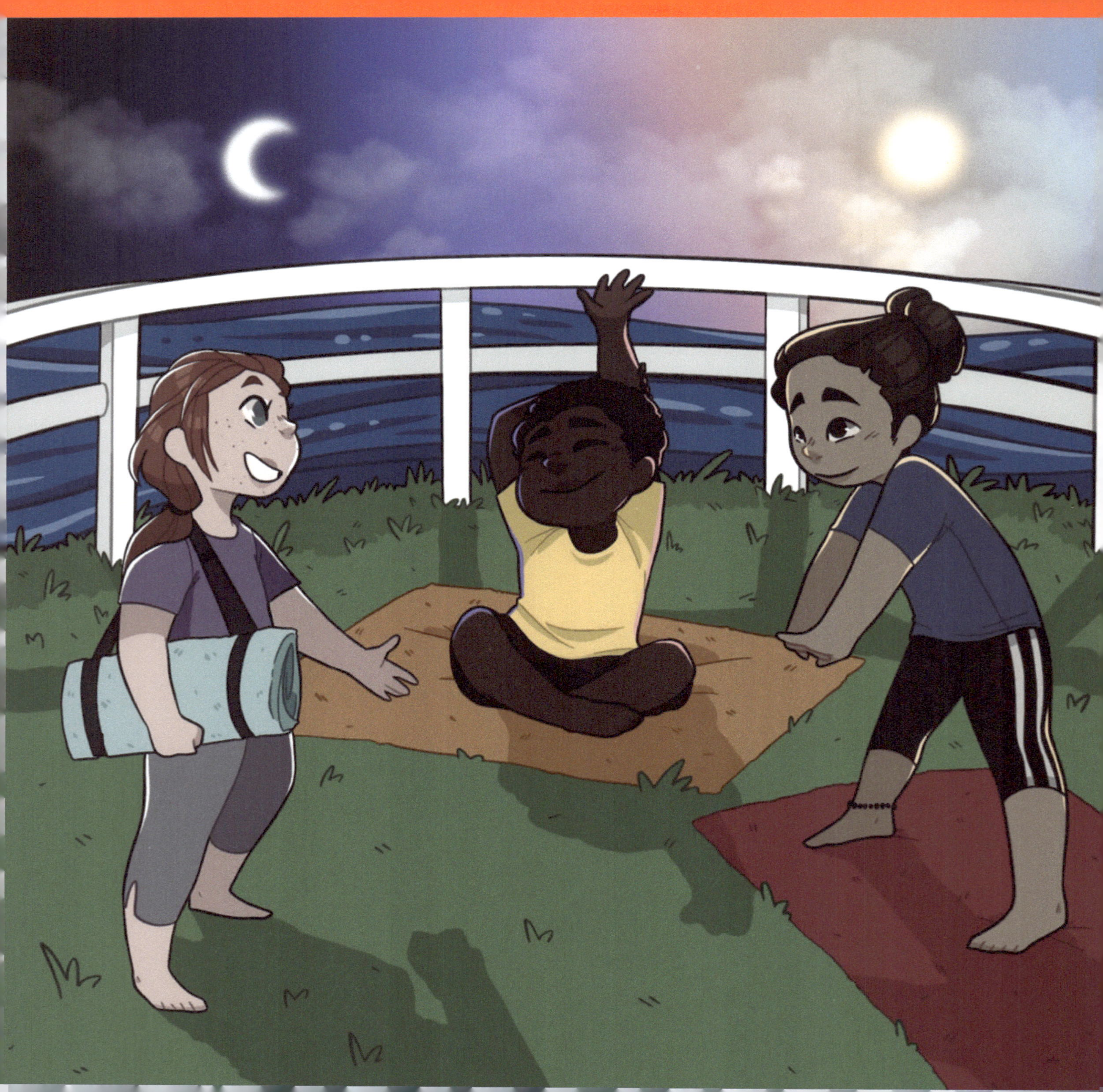

The light within you shows who you are. When you are shining brightly you will go far!

The first pose is the warrior.
So plant your feet firmly to
the ground and say

"I am safe. I am enough!"

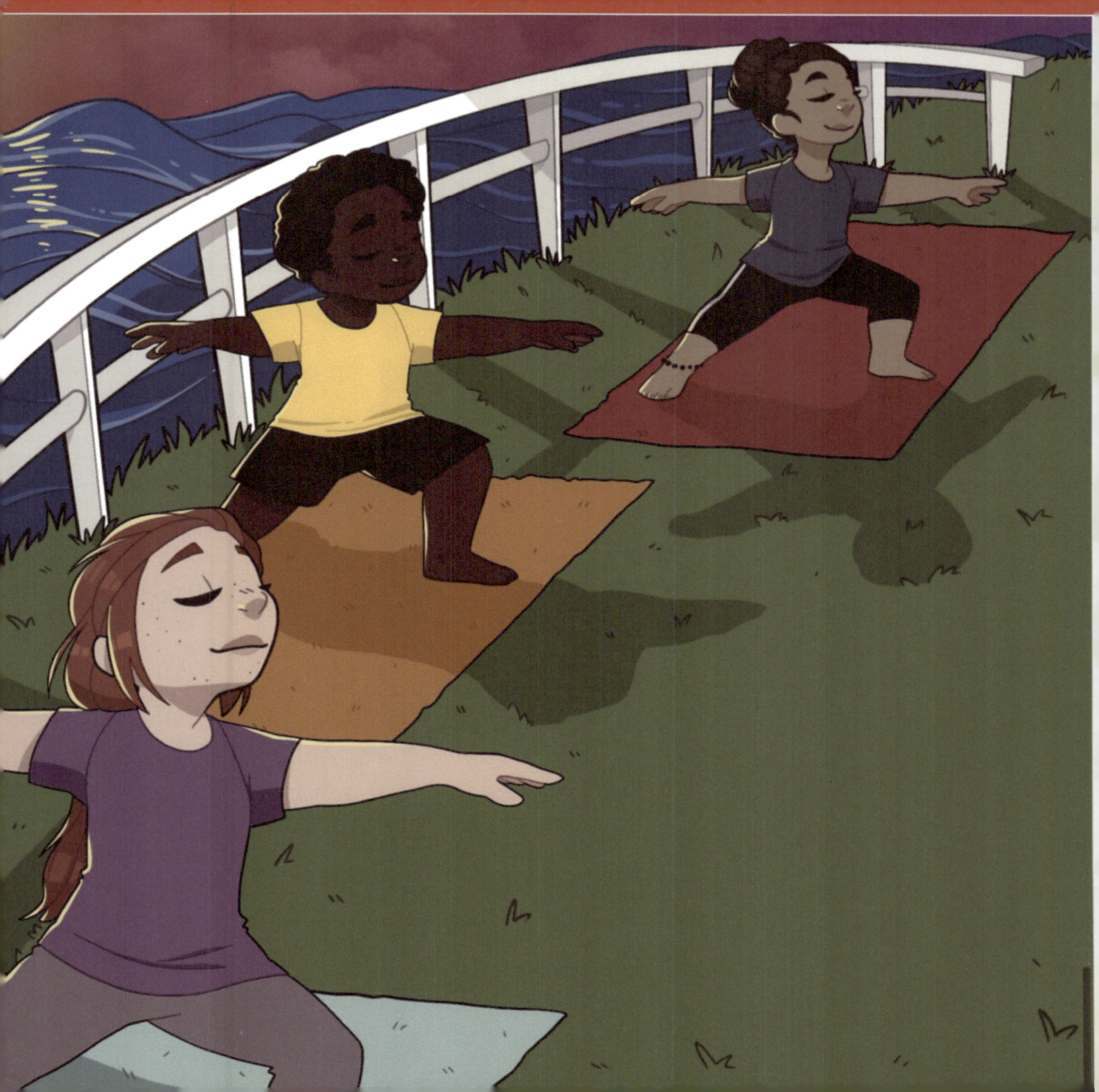

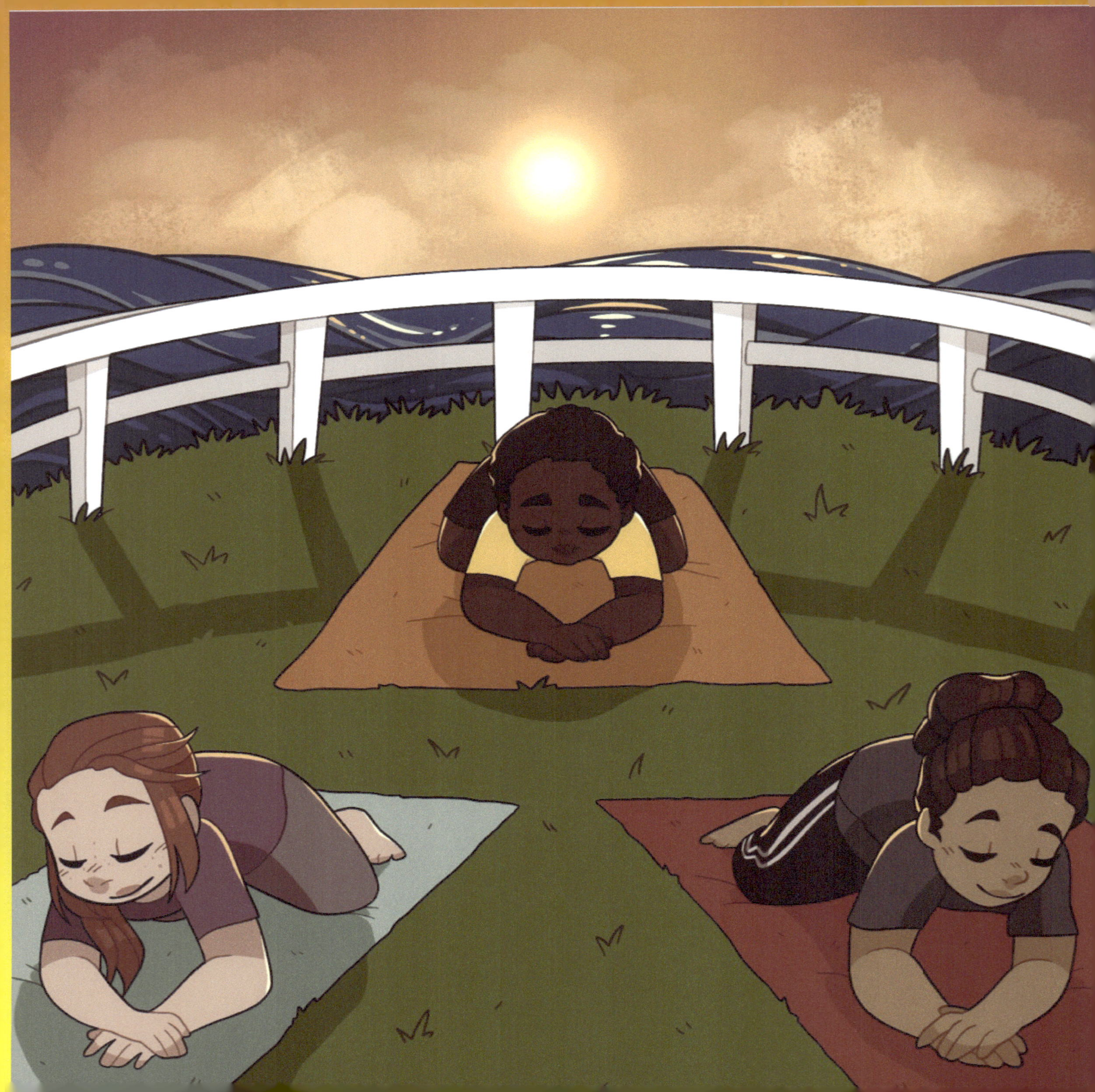

Slowly move to the floor for cow pose with your back rounded. Then drop your back for cat pose.

"I am creative, I enjoy being me"

Roll over and grab your knees for Rock pose. Give yourself a big squeeze.

"I am courageous, I am brave"

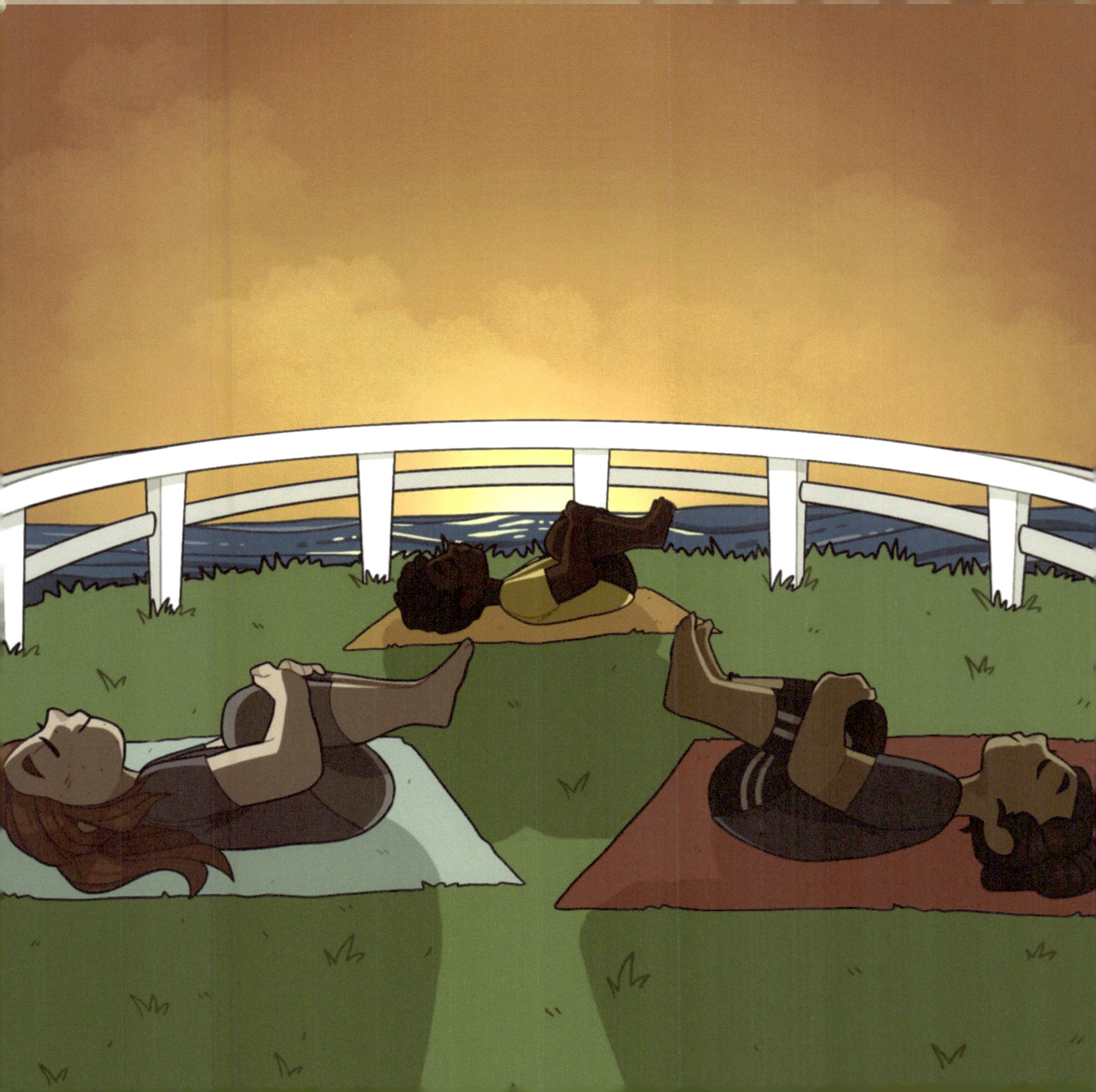

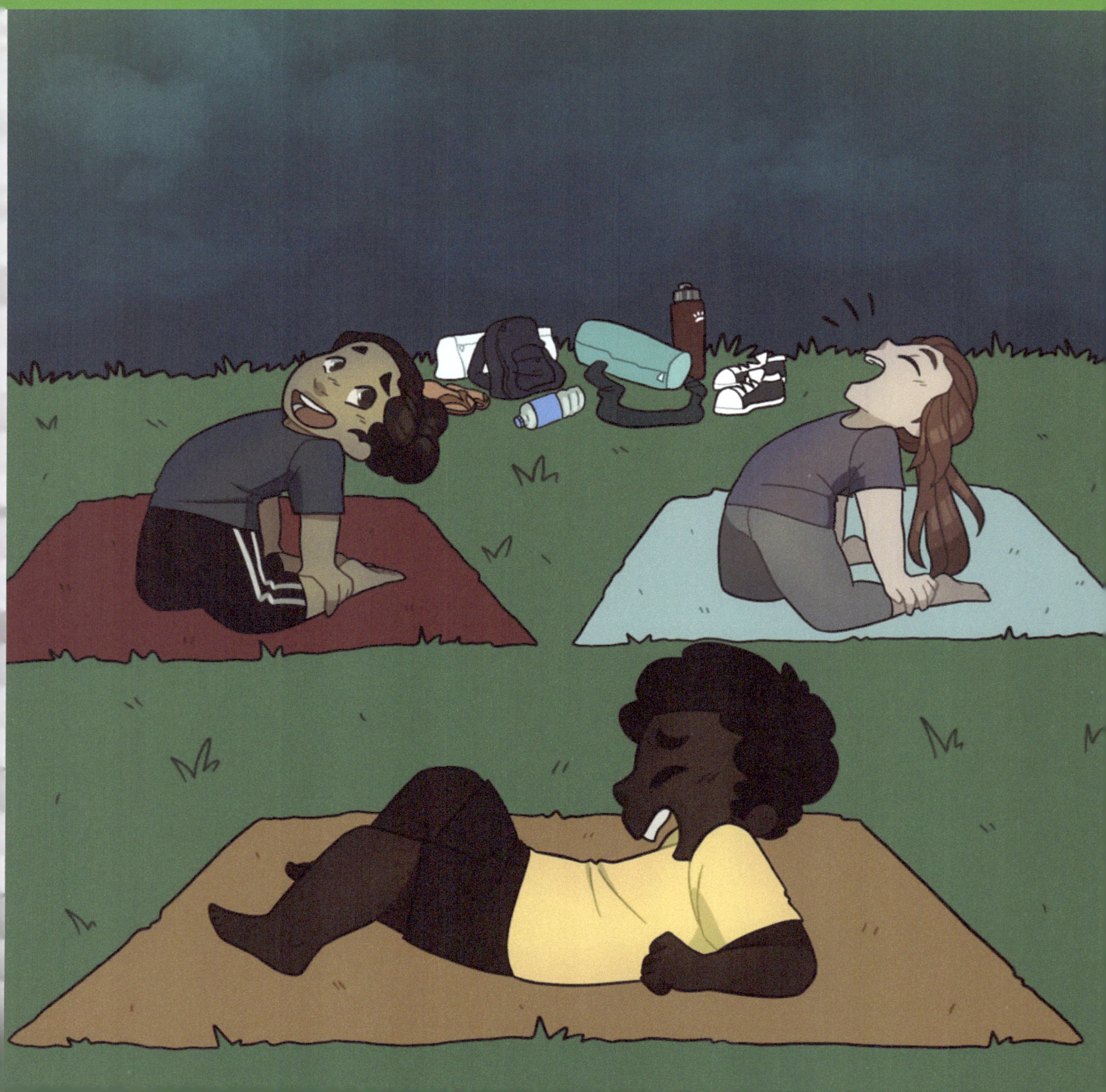

Sit up on your knees, reach back to grab your ankles for camel pose. "I accept myself, I respect myself"

Lean forward and stick
your tongue out. Roar
like a lion!!
"I speak the truth, My
voice is clear"

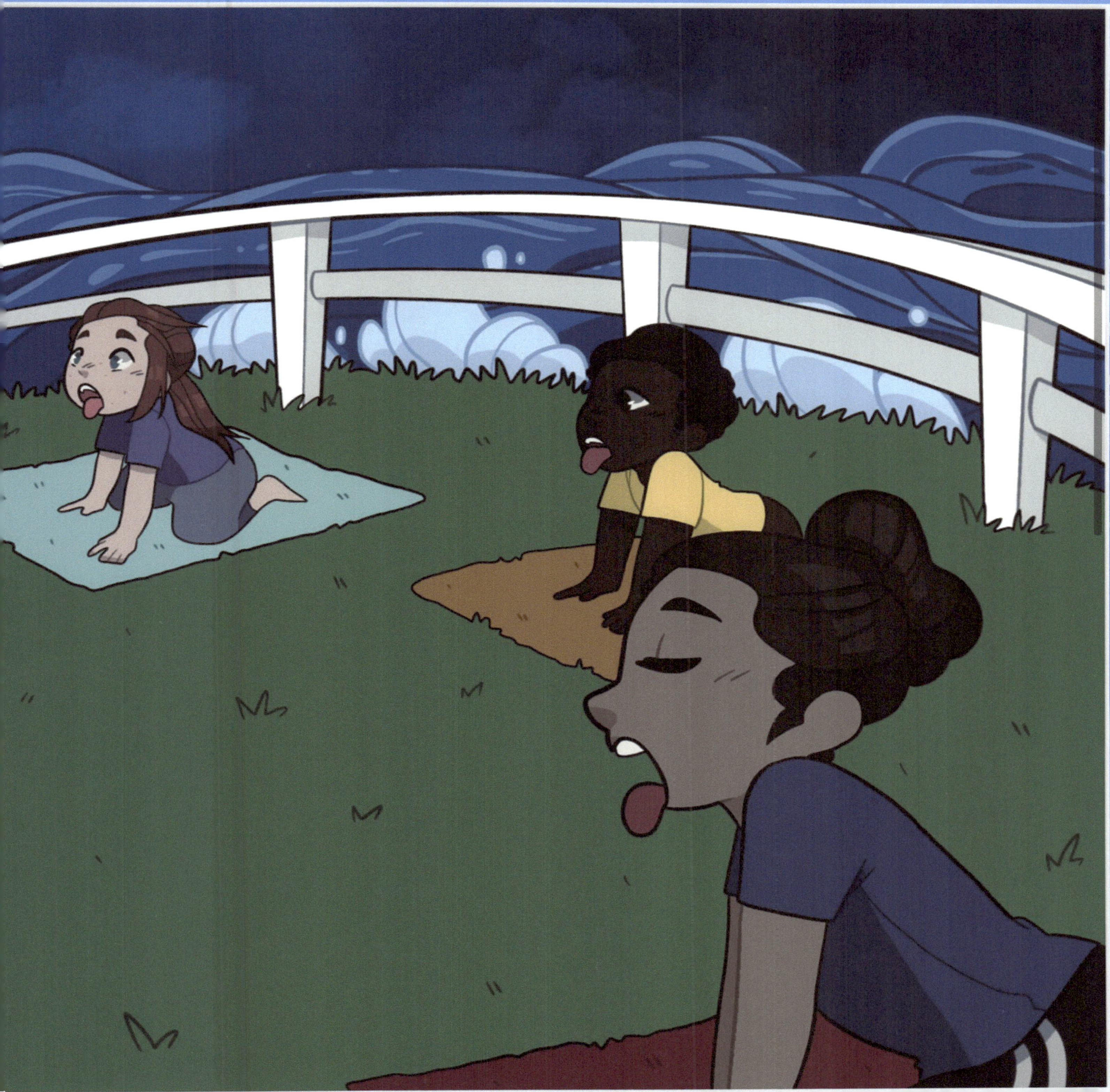

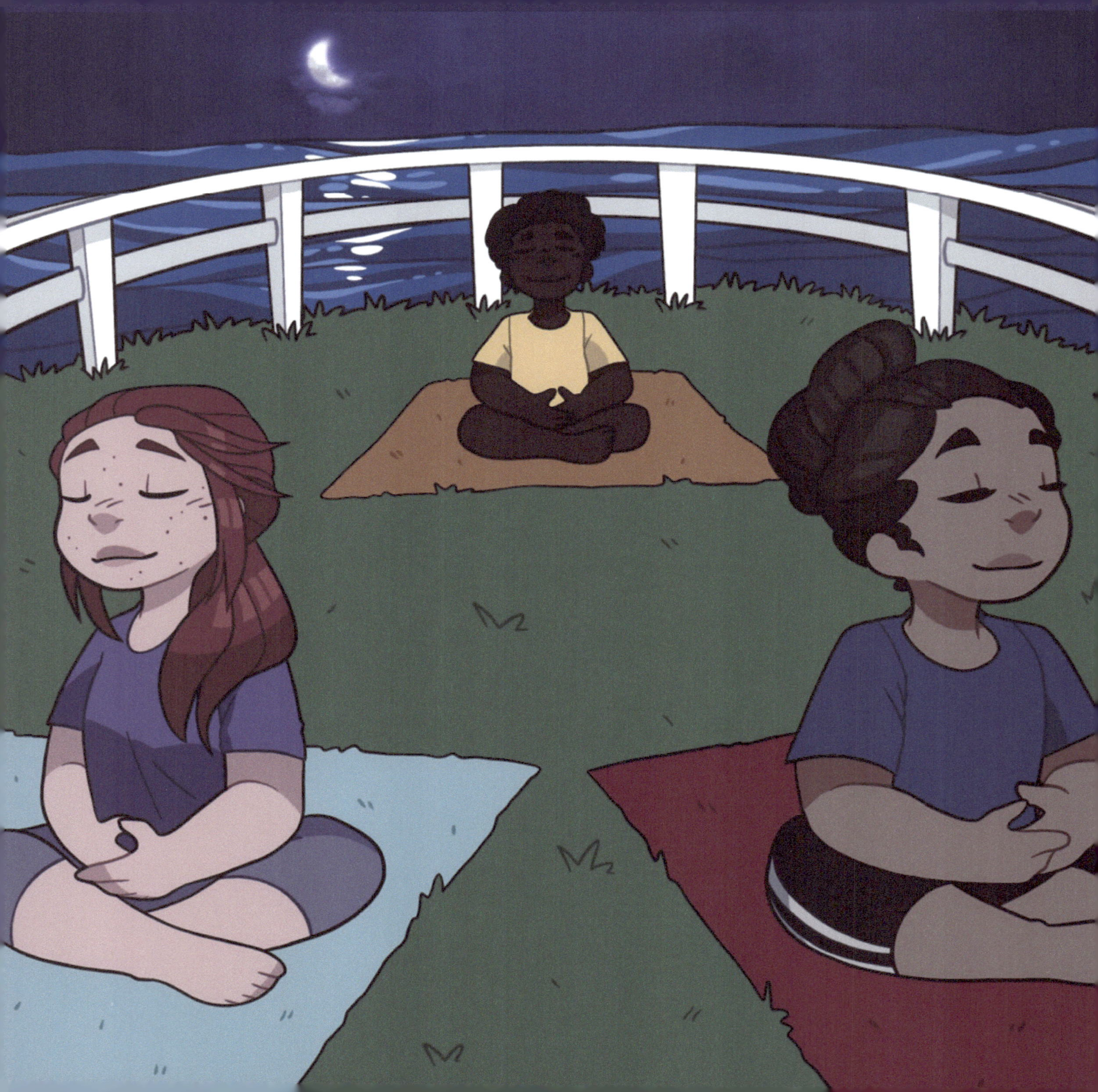

Now we sit as calm as can be. Take a deep breath, in your nose and out your mouth. "I think and see clear"

Stand up and fix your
crown as we stand tall
like the trees.
"All is well and I am at
peace"

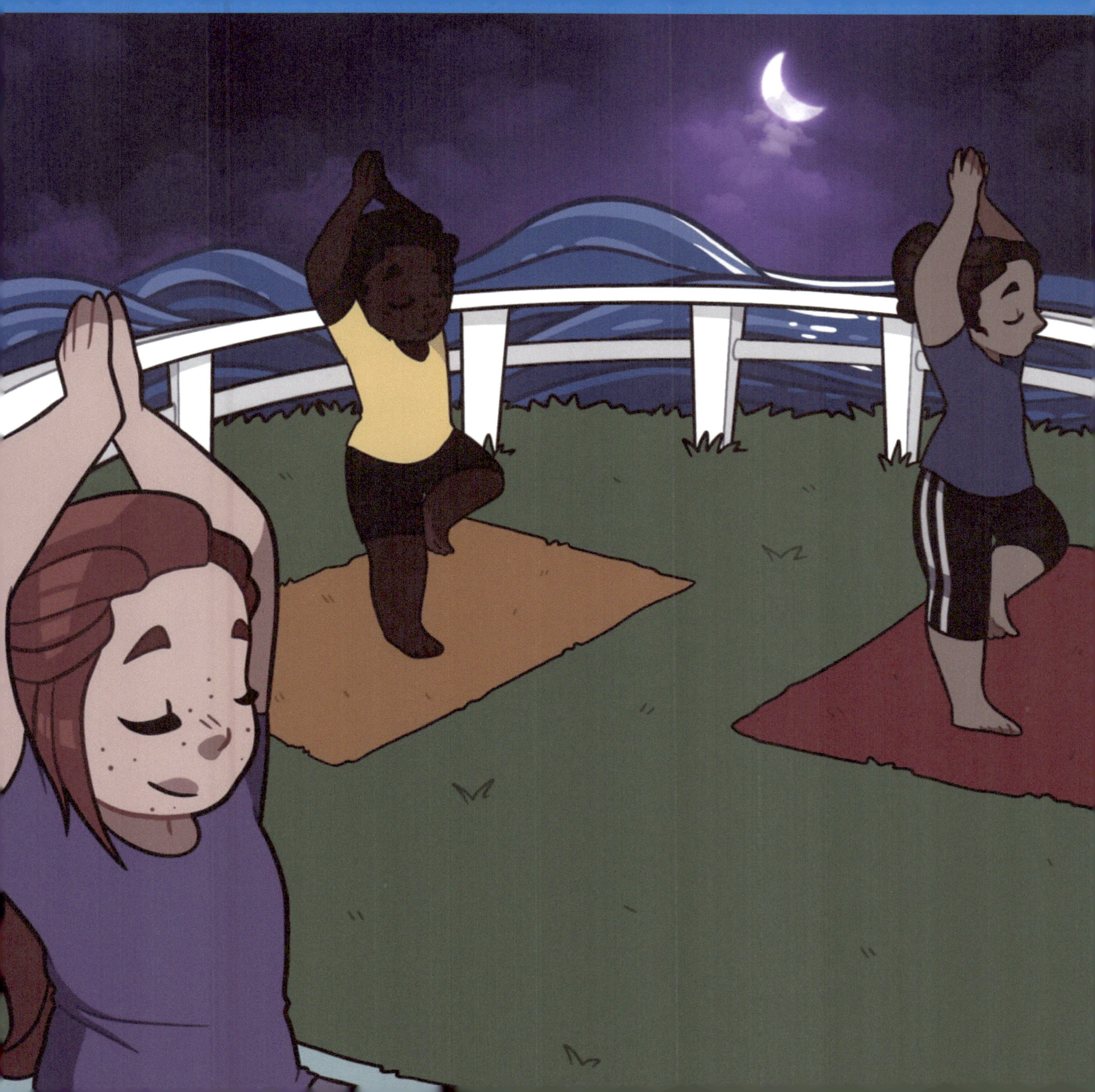

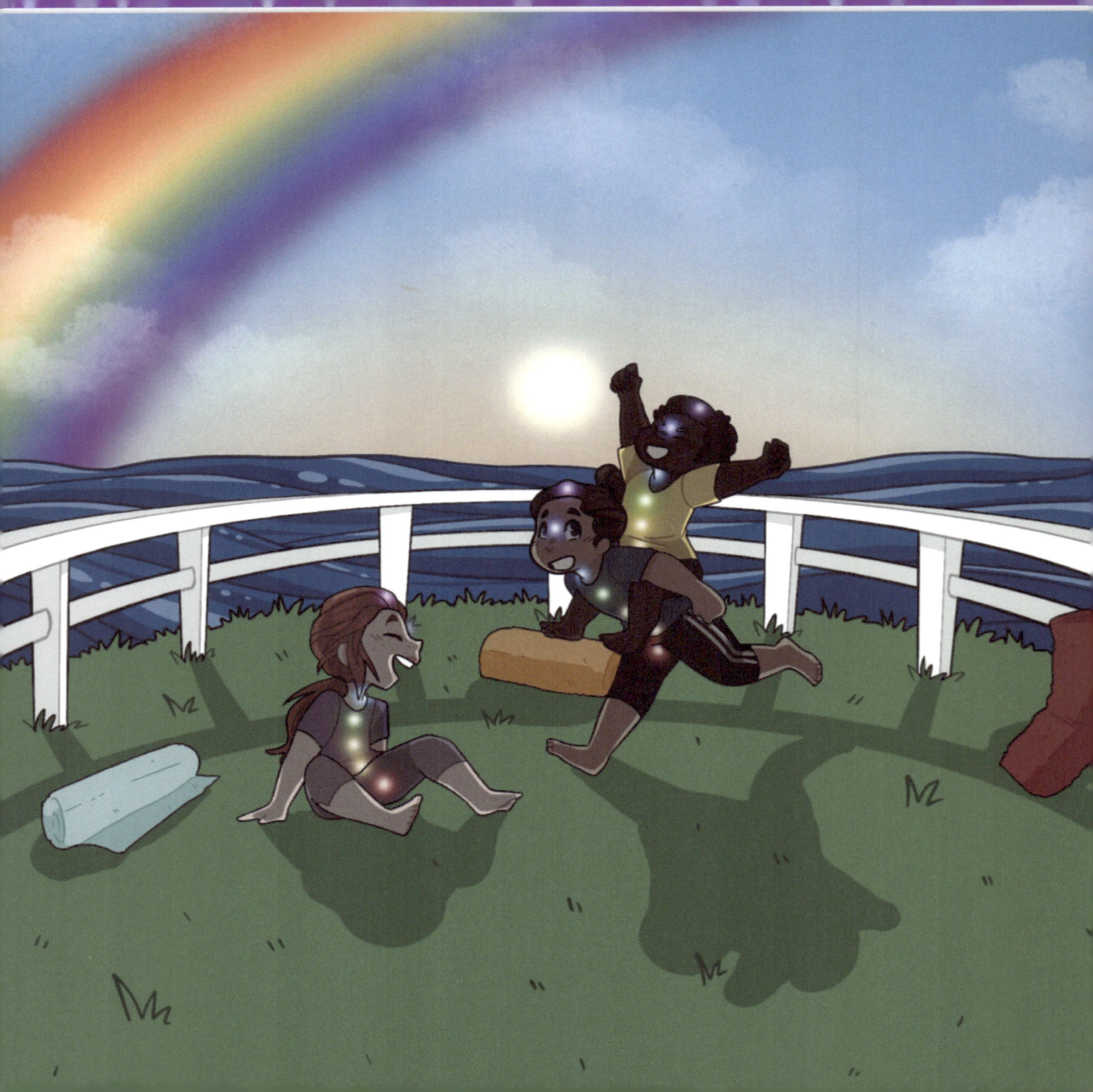

Now that you're aligned, stand up and let's shine! Red, Orange, yellow, Green, Blue. These colors are for me, these colors are for you. "I am unique, I am enough!"

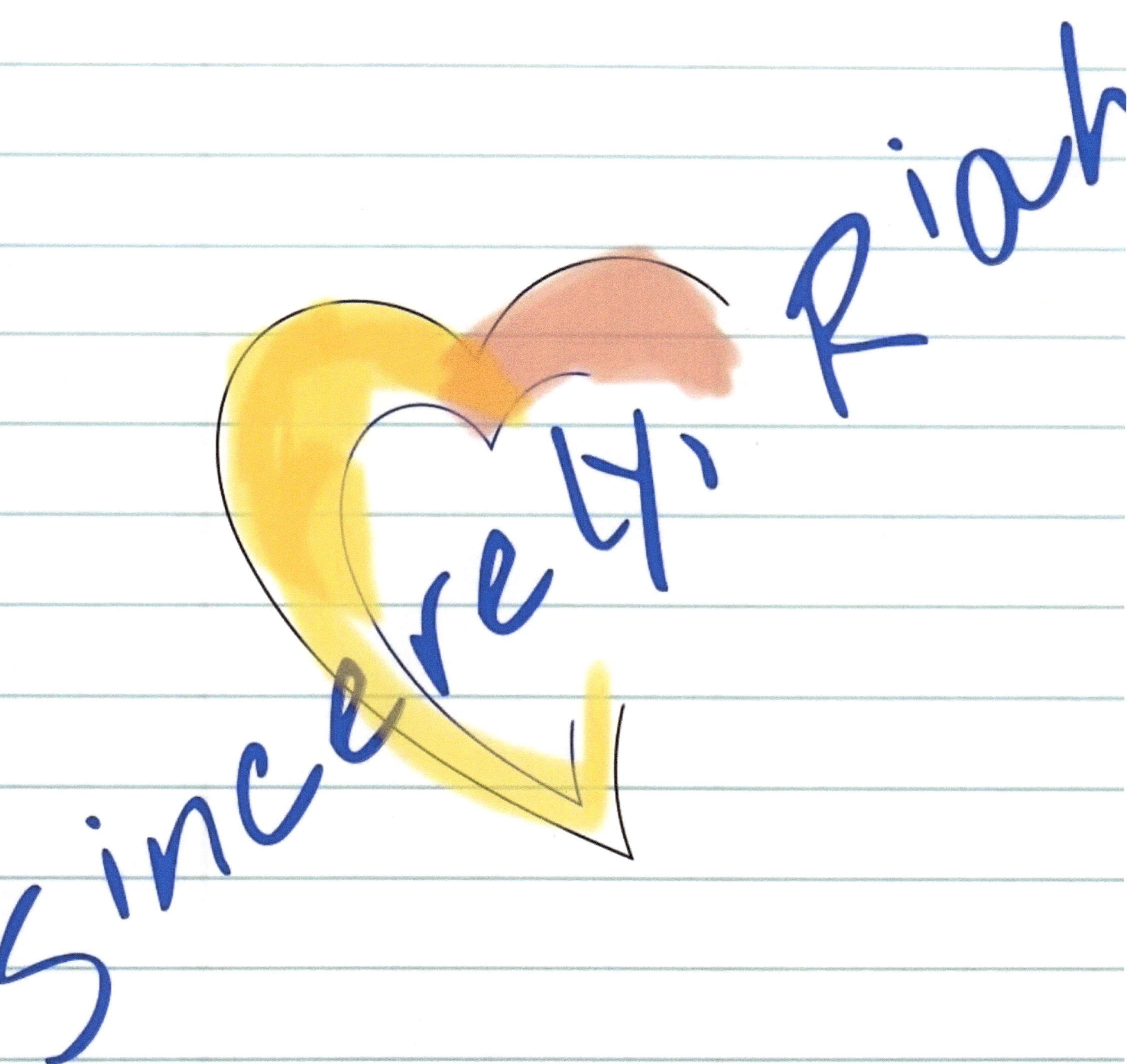

sincerely, Riah